- *Dr. Sebi* -

Cure for Herpes

By **A. J. Bridgeford**

Book 2 of 7: of the series "Dr. Sebi's Natural Remedies"

About the author

A. J. Bridgeford

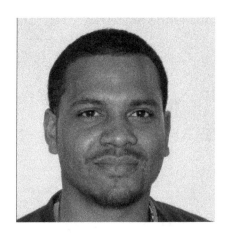

A.J. Bridgeford was born in South Africa and is an incredible traveler who has traveled the globe at least 10 times to discover the wonderful cultures belonging to various countries.

His journey was interrupted when he lost his mother due to an unexpected and terrible illness.

After this happened, he suffered a lot from depression until he realized that his mission was to find a solution to the most well-known diseases and help people in need.

This research led him to Honduras, where he learned and practiced the revolutionary methodologies of the great Dr. Sebi.

Since then, his mission has become to disseminate these incredible treatments and work in the field to improve people's lives.

He is still fighting disease thanks to his private clinics with exceptional results. He wanted to bring back some of his most important knowledge in the field of "alkaline-based medicine" with this book.

With the wish for a healthier life, he reported a quote:

"Life is around us, and we are the fruit of life. Like any fruit, we need the natural elements that the earth makes available to us to become ripe and begin to new life".

Table of Contents

Introduction

In today's world, where everything has almost achieved its highest level of advancement, medical sciences are turning its focus towards nature. Turning towards nature means that people are now relying more on organic herbs and food items. Dr. Sebi's method of curing illnesses or any other disease is purely dependent on an alkaline diet and herbs that possess medicinal benefits. Also, his claim is that all sorts of diseases originate from mucus and acidity in the body; that's why he reinforces eating alkaline food products. Although the number of permitted food items is low still you can make the most of those ingredients by trying and experimenting with new recipes. Other than that, he believes in the cleansing and detoxification of the human body at the most basic level that is the cell. All the toxins that have been built in the body throughout all these years of life, they need to be omitted from the body so that a person can attain the maximum level of better health. Dr. Sebi's methods of curing disease are simple and basic. You have to be determined to adapt to that lifestyle, which Dr. Sebi emphasizes. Herpes is a viral disease and can spread through sexual encounters and other such activities. Through Dr. Sebi's diet, a person can improve and strengthen his immune system so that it is difficult for any sort of microbes to invade the human body systems and cause illness.

Chapter 1: Introduction to Dr. Sebi Treatments and Cures

In this chapter, you will learn about the basics of Dr. Sebi's diet. I have explained in-depth about the benefits of the diet suggested by him. Also, this chapter focuses on the main components, ingredients, and food items of the diet suggested by Dr. Sebi. I have listed down all the fruits, vegetables, herbs, seasonings, oils, and fats. You can easily pick the ingredients from these lists to prepare a meal for yourself. This chapter highlights the main rules to follow the diet designed by Dr. Sebi. These are the strict rules that must be followed and that are to eliminate all the dairy and meat products from the diet, only allowed foods can be consumed, seedless fruits or vegetables cannot be eaten by a person following this diet.

1.1 What is a diet by Dr. Sebi?

Sebi believed that the illness is the product of acidity & mucus in the body, & concluded that in the alkaline climate, infections could not occur. His regimen, which requires a rather rigorous diet and costly medications, promises to detoxify and return alkalinity to the body of the disease (no scientific evidence is sufficient to verify his statements).

The lifestyle limits every form of animal products and, overall, insists on vegan food, but with far more stringent guidelines. It limits seedless fruits, for instance, and only allows Sebi's authorized list of "organic rising grains."

1.2 Food Inventory Dr. Sebi-Recommended Dietary Guide

Vegetable List of Dr. Sebi

Dr. Sebi kept the view that citizens can consume non-GMO diets, as in all the electrical diets. This entails vegetables and fruit rendered seedless or changed to include more minerals and vitamins than they normally do. The selection of vegetables from Dr. Sebi is very wide and varied, with lots of choices for preparing multiple dynamic meals. Included in this category are:

- Arame
- Wild Arugula
- Amaranth

- Bell Pepper

- Garbanzo Beans

- Avocado

- Dandelion Greens

- Cherry and Plum Tomato

- Dulse

- Chayote

- Izote flower and leaf

- Olives

- Kale

- Nopales

- Hijiki

- Lettuce except for iceberg

- Cucumber

- Mushrooms except for Shitake

- Tomatillo

- Nori

- Purslane Verdolaga

- Okra

- Onions

- Watercress

- Sea Vegetables

- Turnip Greens

- Squash

- Zucchini

- Wakame

Fruit List of Dr. Sebi

The fruit range is much more limited, whereas the vegetable list is respectably large, though certain kinds of fruits really aren't permitted to be eaten whilst on the Sebi diet. The fruit category, though, also provides a broad range of choices for diet adherents. For starters, except for cranberries that are a human-made fruit, all berries types are permitted on the Sebi product list. Also, the list contains:

- Bananas

- Dates

- Berries

- Prunes

- Apples

- Cherries

- Melons

- Currants

- Figs

- Soursops

- Grapes

- Mango

- Orange

- Soft Jelly Coconuts

- Papayas

- Plums

- Peaches

- Cantaloupe

- Prickly Pear

- Pears

- Limes

- Tamarind

- Raisins

Dr. Sebi Food List Spices and Seasonings

- Cloves

- Achiote

- Bay Leaf

- Onion Powder

- Cayenne

- Dill

- Sea Salt

- Habanero

- Sweet Basil

- Thyme

- Oregano

- Sage

- Granulated Seaweed Powdered

- Savory

- Tarragon

- Basil

- Alkaline Grains

- Amaranth

- Tef

- Kamut

- Rye

- Wild Rice

- Quinoa

- Spelt

- Fonio

Alkaline Sugars and Sweeteners

- 100% Agave Syrup of cactus

- Date Sugar made with dried dates

Herbal Teas by Dr. Sebi

- Red Raspberry

- Burdock

- Fennel

- Tila

- Elderberry

- Chamomile

- Ginger

Nuts & Seeds

- Brazil Nuts

- Walnuts

- Raw Sesame Seeds

- Hemp seeds

Oils

- Coconut Oil

- Olive Oil

- Hempseed Oil

- Grapeseed Oil

- Avocado Oil

- Sesame Oil

1.3 Diet Rules

1. Its not really advised if the product isn't even in the "dietary Checklist."

2. You must consume 1 gallon a day of fresh spring water.

3. Some medications from Dr. Sebi must be taken one hour prior to "pharmaceuticals."

4. Every item of Dr. Sebi can even be consumed together without any interference.

5. Rigid adherence (consistent with complementary products) to the "dietary Map" offers the best outcomes for disease reversal.

6. It is not acceptable to eat animal foods, hybrid crops, seedless fruits, canned fruits, or alcohol.

7. Using a microwave would "destroy the meal," as per Sebi, so quit using it.

Nutritional Guide by Dr. Sebi-Mucus Lowering Alkaline Diet

This mucus lowering alkaline diet that is made from non-modified alkalizing foods from plant origin is influenced by Dr. Sebi.

The acidic concentration throughout the body that defends against unhealthy mucus production that harms organs & contributes to disease growth is regulated by these foods.

Following the dietary guide from Dr. Sebi will give you the contentment.

Eventually, wean yourself out of meat until you start following an alkaline vegetarian diet and just consume fish as well as a tiny portion of dairy. At the starting point, only eat some ice-cream and yogurt every now and then.

In no time, you will see yourself by being a meat lover to a total vegetarian. You will notice the elevating amounts of energy in your body by eliminating meat from the diet.

Adopting Through Dr. Sebi's Alkaline Diet

Dr. Sebi that used his "African-Bio Mineral Equilibrium" to improve wellness and strength. His approach included the usage of a pure alkaline plant-based diet & herbs so that to alkalize the system and restore the alkalinity of the body and homeostasis.

Only organic alkaline fruits, vegetables, nuts, grains, and legumes were used in the diet, which would alkalize & extract mucus from the body.

He often used organic alkaline herbs along with the diet to disinfect the cells of the body at the cellular level & intra-cellular grade.

The alkaline diet has been built on the idea in an acidic setting; illness can only occur. The body acts to establish a 7.4 pH state throughout the blood that is mildly alkaline.

The bloodstream is the homeostasis site of equilibrium, and the bloodstream can lend alkaline compounds & minerals from the bones & fluids across the bloodstream as the body gets too acidic to bring them into the blood and maintain its pH stable.

This threatens the wellbeing of multiple body parts & leads to the stimulation of illnesses.

Approach for Disease by Dr. Sebi

Dr. Sebi's response to sickness is sickness:

Finds the genesis where even mucous membrane has been damaged & when. For e.g., where there is excessive mucous membrane in bronchial passages, Bronchitis is the disease; Pneumonia is the disease if this is in the lungs; Diabetes seems to be in the pancreas; Arthritis is in the joints.

Dr. Sebi utilized alkaline products & alkaline extracts have been used by several herbal professionals as part of the alkaline food listings that are distributed across the internet.

Dr. Sebi adopted common medicinal herbs that disinfect the blood & disinfect the stomach, such as dandelion, sarsaparilla, & burdock root. These herbs are now extensively used by common and-holistic wellness initiatives.

Since the early '90s, Dr. Sebi had used his alkaline technique and considering him to be a founder in that same alkaline diet trend.

Centered on Dr. Sebi's food list, create a list of foods & herbs could use. (Dr. Sebi recommended avoiding having something that was not mentioned in the diet guide.)

It is unbelievable the manner that an alkaline diet helps you perform. The amount of energy will be great, and you will not feel exhausted anymore, except during the hectic days.

You would think that you will be going to miss consuming tuna, but you should not really be worried about consuming it anymore. You will start reducing weight & it would sound like you are not holding any sort of dead weight. You will be sleeping deeply now, and then when you are awake, you will be wide awake straight away & completely awake all day long.

Approach to Consuming by Dr. Sebi

Spring Water

It is important to drink lots of water per day to make the alkaline diet function. Dr. Sebi recommends consuming a gallon of that spring water per day, & almost the same quantity is recommended by health organizations.

The mature body is made of 70 percent water. To work properly, all the physiological processes of the body require sufficient volumes of water. Water reduces the body's toxins, cushions your joints & organs, as well as helps in nutrient absorption.

Some of the herbs that Dr. Sebi recommends are diuretics that eliminate contaminants from the body and improve urination. In order to help the proper working of the body, you must substitute water.

Spring water occurs naturally as alkaline water & the hydration & organic proportion of electrolytes are better assisted.

Microwaving is not advised by Dr. Sebi's diet guide since it affects the nutrients of the food.

You will also encounter contrasting evidence on whether microwaving harms food nutrients, including research that confirms both sides. You must choose to never microwave the food since it is unhealthy.

Try to avoid warming your food at all and consume raw food because heating up the food, whether its oven or burner, will damage the nutrients present in the food.

Dr. Sebi would not suggest that you consume items that do not exist on Dr. Sebi's diet guide.

Dr. Sebi's product list is very narrow & lacks several plant-based whole-food products.

Dr. Sebi advises that hybrid foods (crops & their fruits rendered by unusually cross-pollinating 2 or even more plants) be discouraged because, to their disadvantage, they alter the genetic form, electrical composition, & pH equilibrium.

Garlic, the plant food that we are used to consuming and is not really the safest product to consume, is one such product.

Chapter 2: Where Herpes Came From?

In this chapter, the details about herpes are mentioned. The details include all types and signs and symptoms of this viral disease. There are also preventive measures that can help prevent the disease. This is contagious and can be spread through touch as well. The most common type of it is oral herpes, where lesions appear around the mouth and, in worst-case scenarios, can spread all over the face as well. So the safety measures that I have mentioned should be followed to avoid the contact of this viral disease.

2.1 What's Herpes?

It is indeed a virus that might stay inactive or allow the body to undergo the flare-up. Two major strains are known.

While the herpes virus group has eight variants, including the Epstein-Barr virus, here we will concentrate on the two most prevalent types of HSV.

HSV-1, or oral herpes, is a type of herpes spread by saliva. During infancy or adulthood, many persons with oral herpes were possibly compromised by exchanging a straw, cup, eating utensils, toothbrush, gum, or kissing.

Among the most prevalent sexual diseases is HSV-2, also identified for genital herpes. The incidents involving genital herpes within that U.S. are above 1 in 6 people aged 14-49, as per the CDC. In women, it is often around twice as high as in males.

2.2 The Symptoms of Herpes

In the mouth as well as on and across the lips, HSV-1 or oral herpes may trigger fever blisters or cold sores. Rectal & genital blisters can also be induced by it.

Herpetic lesions or Blisters or may also develop around the rectum, genitals, & mouth because of HSV-2. They cause blisters, which can last 7 days – 4 weeks to recover as these lesions split open. Additional signs could be:

• A burning feeling when urinating

• Poor odor discharge from genitalia

• Bleeding in women between cycles

Symptoms that precede an epidemic, such as:

- Pain in the vagina

- Numbness or Shooting pain in the hips, butt, or legs

They must have some flu-like effects after the infectious individual's first epidemic, such as:

- Headaches

- Aches in the body

- Fever

- Inflamed lymph nodes

As the infection remains with them forever, individuals with genital herpes can experience multiple outbreaks throughout their lifetime, until adequately handled with traditional herpes medication. Consequent breakouts over time might be less extreme.

It is often normal to have little or no signs, or just moderate symptoms, in individuals with genital or oral herpes. Many persons who bear this type of virus may not really realize that they have it. This is due to the sores hat tare confused for a specific skin condition, including a zit or the ingrown hair, or they have no effects.

2.3 What triggers herpes, & how does it get passed on?

From saliva, HSV-1 or oral herpes is transmitted. HSV-1 can be spread to the genitals during oral sex and induce the genital HSV-1 outbreak.

Via interaction with genital secretions, herpes blisters, & mucosal surfaces, HSV-2 or genital herpes is spread. Both viruses can also be released from skin or mucosa that do not tend to have signs or to be contaminated.

The individual must refrain from oral, anal, or vaginal sex with someone who is affected with HSV-2 to avoid contractions with genital herpes. To do this, you should refrain from sex entirely, or just have sex in a legally monogamous partnership in which neither spouse exhibits genital herpes.

The use of contraceptives might even minimize the risk of genital herpes, but lesions could be present in places that are not covered by condoms, and no lesions need to be visible for the disease to spread. Some strategies to avoid or minimize the transmission of the infection can involve taking medicine each day to avoid an epidemic, or after an epidemic, avoiding participating in anal, oral, or vaginal intercourse.

2.4 What's the distinction between oral herpes & genital herpes?

Many people are uncertain as to what to name these diseases, and that there occur 2 distinct forms of herpes viruses, which are HSV-1 & HSV-2, that may exist on multiple body sections. But it's pretty easy actually:

It's labeled genital herpes anytime you either have HSV-1 or 2 on or near your vulva, vagina, butt, cervix, scrotum, penis, anus, inner thighs).

It's labeled oral herpes anytime you either have HSV-1 or 2 in or near your mouth, lips & throat. Fever blisters or Cold sores are often called oral herpes.

HSV-1 tends to cause oral herpes, & genital herpes is typically induced by HSV-2, with each strain choosing to reside in its favorite location. But with all forms of herpes, able to infect a region is entirely probable. For starters, when somebody having a cold sore over their lips offers you oral sex, you might develop HSV-1 over your genitals. And when you provide oral sex, someone having HSV-2 over their genitals, you will develop HSV-2 on the mouth.

2.5 How do you develop herpes?

Through skin-to-skin touch with anyone who got the infection, herpes can quickly be transmitted. You will get it, typically through anal, oral, & vaginal intercourse, anytime your mouth or genitals meet their mouth and/or genitals.

Herpes may be spread even though the mouth, anus, or vagina does not reach out all path into the tongue or penis. To propagate herpes, you don't need to cum. All that it takes seems to be some simple contact of skin. Kissing anyone that got oral herpes will even cause you to get herpes.

You will quickly infect the skin of your mouth, eyes, & genitals. If there's a path for herpes to get through, such as by a wound, rash, burn, or other infections, other skin areas may get contaminated. In order to get herpes, you may not have to have intercourse. Herpes may also be spread in non-sexual contexts, such as whether you are pecked on the lips by a parent with the cold sore. While they were children, most individuals having oral herpes developed it. While vaginal childbirth, a mother may transfer herpes to the new-born, but that's very uncommon.

If you tap herpes sore and touch your genitals, eyes, or mouth without washing the hands first, you will transmit herpes to any other areas of your body. This way, you will even move herpes onto somebody else.

Herpes is more common when the sores are exposed and moist since the infection is quickly transmitted by fluid through herpes blisters. Although if there have been no sores, herpes may still "shed" & get passed on to someone, and the skin appears perfectly fine.

The majority of people receive herpes through someone who has no sores at all. Without showing some signs, it will remain in the body for a long time, but it is impossible to tell for certain how and where you caught it. That's why it's a pretty sly virus that so many individuals have herpes.

You can't catch herpes by hugging, shaking hands, sneezing, coughing, or using toilet seats because the infection dies rapidly outside of the body.

2.6 Who's at risk of getting diseases of herpes simplex?

Anyone, irrespective of age, maybe contaminated by HSV. Almost exclusively, the probability is dependent on susceptibility to the virus.

Individuals are increasingly at risk in instances of sexual transmission HSV because they have intercourse that is not covered by contraceptives or other protective techniques.

Some HSV-2 risk factors include:

• Having several sex partners

• Physical intercourse at an earlier age

• Female being

• Getting another virus spread via sex

• Possession of a compromised immune system

When a pregnant lady has a genital herpes infection at the period of delivery, the infant will be subjected to both forms of HSV and will be at risk of severe complications.

2.7 What is the future regarding herpes simplex in the long-term?

For the remainder of their life, individuals who get contaminated from HSV may have the infection. The infection can continue to exist in the nerve cells of an infected individual, although it doesn't show symptoms.

Frequent outbreaks can occur in certain persons. After they have become bitten, some can only undergo one infection, and afterward, the virus might be inactive. And if a strain is inactive, an infection may be caused by such triggers. They include:

• Stress

• Menstruation cycles

• Fever or disease

• Exposure to the rays or sunburn

Over time, it is suspected that occurrence -become less frequent when the body continues to produce antibodies.

There are normally no risks if a typically stable individual is afflicted with infection.

2.8 Preventing the transmission of diseases with herpes simplex

While there is no treatment for herpes, you should take precautions to discourage or avoid the spread of HSV to some other person from transmitting the virus.

If you have an HSV-1 epidemic, try taking just a few protective steps:

• Try preventing overt physical interaction with many other persons.

• Don't exchange certain things such as towels, cups, clothes, silverware, lip balm, or makeup, which can transmit the virus out.

• In an occurrence, do not partake in sexual contact, kissing, or some such form of sexual interaction.

• To avoid contact with lesions, clean your hands well & use medicine using cotton swabs.

During a disease, individuals with HSV-2 can prevent some form of sexual contact with the other persons. A contraceptive must be used through sex if the individual is not having signs but has also been confirmed having the virus. However, the infection may also be transmitted from exposed skin to a mate, including while using the contraceptive.

To keep the pathogen from harming their new-born infants, people who are expecting & contaminated might just have to use medication.

Chapter 3: How to Cure Herpes with Dr. Sebi Treatments

This chapter will give you a complete insight into what is detoxification and cleansing and what is the difference between them and in what context they are used interchangeably. There are more than one approaches to detoxify the body. Basic steps towards cleansing or detoxification include limiting alcohol, be physically active, get enough and sound sleep, consume fresh and organic food items, try to avoid processed food items. According to the results required, there are different types of detox diets that are being used. A few of the major disadvantages of detoxification are dehydration, deficiency of certain nutrients, and digestive problems.

3.1 Detoxification and Cleansing

As strategies to remove pollutants from the body, reduce weight, or improve wellbeing, a number of "detoxification" foods, regimens, & treatments, also called "detoxes" or "cleanses," have been introduced.

The words cleanse & detox are also used synonymously, and although both eliminate contaminants from the body, two separate items are a detox as well as cleanse. It is clean at the core of the term "cleanse," and you must think of washing as a way to clean the body. In order to specifically remove toxins, cleanse frequently utilizes vitamins or tablets, and cleanses typically concentrate mostly on the digestive system. Detox services, on the other side, aim to help the normal toxin-eliminating cycles in the body. Because the liver & the kidneys are the key detoxing centers in the body, successful detox programs concentrate on helping the kidneys and liver through supplying them with the vitamins and nutrients they have to operate optimally.

What are poisons anyway, then? Heavy metals are top of the mind, like arsenic, but chronic chemical contaminants, chemicals, & pesticides are still included in the report. Toxins are simply toxic compounds that will reside in the bloodstream, disturbing cells, triggering irritation, & interacting with the usual functions of the body.

Indications of toxins or a heavy toxin load (and hence the need for detoxification or cleansing) provide the following:

- fatigue

- headaches

- joint pain

- depression

- anxiety

- constipation

3.2 The cleansing journey

Making the stomach safe is linked with cleansing. The digestive system is the system the body receives its nutrients from. It becomes inefficient in performing out its tasks as it gets unstable. In the stomach, the pile-up of the dump will turn poisonous, contributing to pain and disease. Bloating is among the symptoms of a dysfunctional stomach. When the body cannot get rid of waste as it can, that's due to the accumulation of gas. The food continues to decompose then. Food, as meant by default, must be natural and as organic.

There are both positive and destructive microbes in the digestive system. It contributes to problems if the equilibrium of such bacteria is disrupted. Purging, in which a laxative is used to eliminate human waste, parasites, and other such unnecessary material, is the essential method of cleansing. The concern with this technique, though, is that it would be non-selective & clears up the beneficial with the harmful. It may also be harmful since, during the phase, you may lose extra water, which would make you drained. One of its reasons the body system gets a strip of toxic chemicals is to consume lots of water.

A vice president & dietician of the Sports Education Society, Marie Spano, claims that workout and adequate sleep play a vital role in making your function on the detox regimen.

Through curing the gut by taking note of what goes through it, a healthy way to detox is to practice regularly. It's considered fast food, and it doesn't have the nutrition your body requires. Instead, clogging things up appears to screw with the digestive tract. Soy, gluten, dairy, sugar, & caffeine-containing foods can be removed and substituted with unprocessed agricultural substitutes & additives.

The method of cleansing is not only complete with the clearance of waste from the digestive system. By supplying nutritious food that makes the gut function at its peak, it should be cured. This requires balanced food that has adequate nutrition, which tends to maintain the safe levels of microbes in the stomach, such as good bacteria—organic beverages, such as unflavored probiotic yogurt, often aid.

Minneapolis Running's Sara Welle speaks about the advantages she gained as a competitor from the cleansing plan. You must go through a well before-cleanse process for you to start the detox method, where you'll have to strip out alcohol & different highly processed foods. Her program's early days were unpleasant. However, she noticed that her stress levels became much greater as the system matured and began to operate properly.

3.3 The detox route

Another approach to clear the body of destructive chemicals is to detox. Normally, through the liver, skin, and kidneys, the body requires the removal of pollutants.

The contributions of these organs can be strengthened by Detox. So, what toxins are attacked by the process? For example, there are contaminants in the atmosphere you breathe in that make their way through your bloodstream, where they settle and create pain. Chemicals such as toxins, preservatives, & additives are still used in a number of products. During this time, meat must be avoided.

One of the actors whose detox performed with is Gwyneth Paltrow. Over a 21-day duration, it is circulated. It's named The Safe Method by the psychiatrist who developed it. To clear the body of contaminants, he recommends a diet of shakes, nutritious foods, and vitamins—any of his patient's record post-program weight loss.

Your skin is often loaded with a mixture of chemicals hidden on the lotions of creams and other products you use. Often, the organs associated with detoxifying get overloaded. The detox can be supported by ingredients such as lemon, garlic, spinach, pineapple, and ginger. As several may have detrimental consequences, you can address them with a nutritionist. For starters, garlic thins the blood, which may threaten someone whose blood doesn't easily coagulate. Health supplements, too, aid enhance the health of the liver and kidneys.

What are some detoxification/Cleansing approaches?

Many detoxification programs are offered in an integrative health care model. The following areas are some strategies you can follow to eliminate toxins in your body:

- Exercise/movement
- Body-mind balance (yoga, meditation, breathing, prayer)
- Pure/alkaline water
- Diet
- Fasting
- Juicing
- Supplements
- Detox Massages and Body Scrubs
- Infrared Sauna
- Lymphatic Drainage

- Ozonetherapy (autohemotherapy)

- Detox infusions

- Colon Hydrotherapy

- Osteopathy

Why Detoxification/Cleansing?

Practically, there have been 8 ways in which contaminants impact our bodies that need detoxification.

Pollutants poison enzymes such that they don't act correctly.

Our body systems are the engines of enzymes. To generate molecules, create energy, & build cell structures, and physiological response relies on enzymes. Toxins harm enzymes and thereby impair myriad body functions, such as inhibiting haemoglobin development in the blood or reducing the ability of the body to resist free-radical damage, which accelerates aging.

Structural minerals are displaced by pollutants, resulting in weakened bones.

For lifetime mobility, people have to retain good bone density. There is indeed a twofold consequence as toxins replace the calcium contained in the bone: weakened skeletal systems and enhanced toxins, generated through bone degradation, circulated around the body.

Organs are impaired by toxins.

Nearly all the tissues and structures are damaged by toxins. The Toxin Cure, my novel, concentrates primarily on detox organs. Your detoxification can backfire because the body would remain acidic if the digestive system, liver, and kidneys are too contaminated that they are not able to cleanse efficiently.

DNA, which raises the risk of aging & degeneration, is impaired by toxins.

Many widely used contaminants, phthalates, estrogen that are poorly detoxified, and benzene-containing materials damage DNA.

Toxins change the expression of genes.

To respond to shifts in our parts of the body & the outside world, our genes turn off and on. But certain contaminants trigger our DNA in unhealthy ways or block them.

Toxins destroy the membranes of cells such that they do not respond properly.

In cell membranes, "signaling" exists in the body. Harm to such membrane inhibits them from obtaining essential stimuli, such as insulin that does not warn the cells to consume more sugar, or body tissues that do not respond to the magnesium message to relax.

Toxins interact and create imbalances in the hormones.

Toxins trigger chemicals, disrupt, imitate, and destroy them. For example, arsenic disrupts the cells' thyroid hormone receptors because the cells do not obtain the signal through thyroid hormones, which trigger the metabolism to rev up. Inexplicable exhaustion is the consequence.

Toxins, finally, but not only, potentially inhibit the detoxification potential, and it's the worst concern of all.

It's tougher when you're already really unhealthy and have to detoxify urgently, even when you're not unhealthy. In other words, your hard-working cleansing mechanism is more likely to run below average exactly as you will need your recovery systems more (to fix health problems). And why? Since your recovery potential has been exhausted by the strong toxic burden, you still bear. That is right. The more contaminants your body is burdened with, the stronger the harm to the detoxification processes in the body.

That's why it's so an essential challenge to rebuild your detox body parts and your detox mechanisms with them. The net effect is that contaminants will then be freely expelled by the body.

3.4 Helpful Ideas for Detox

While the use of such detox diets to eliminate toxins from the body is not confirmed by current evidence, some changes in diet & lifestyle habits can help reduce the toxin load & support the detoxification mechanism of your body.

Eat foods containing Sulphur. Sulfur-high foods such as broccoli, onions, as well as garlic improve the removal of heavy metals such as mercury.

Try chlorella. As per animal research, chlorella is indeed a form of algae that has several vital nutrients and may boost the absorption of contaminants such as heavy metals.

Using cilantro to spice dishes. Cilantro improves the excretion of many pollutants, including heavy metals such as lead and contaminants such as phthalates & insecticides.

Glutathione Help. Consuming foods high in Sulphur, such as meat, broccoli, & garlic, may increase the role of glutathione, the significant antioxidant the body creates that is strongly engaged in purification.

Turn to cleaning items that are safe. You will reduce your sensitivity to possibly harmful substances by preferring natural cleaning materials like vinegar & baking soda above synthetic cleaning agents.

Choose natural treatment for the body. Your susceptibility to toxins will also be minimized by utilizing natural deodorants, shampoos, cosmetics, moisturizers, as well as other personal care items.

Chapter 4: Recipes Approach to Cure Herpes

As the one who is opting for this type of diet, he or she will think of how little options they are left with. So to ease their problem, I have gathered some delicious and easy recipes in this chapter, which you can prepare and consume at the time. These recipes are rich in nutrients and are closer to nature as well. They have an enormous amount of benefits.

4.1 Pasta Salad Alkaline

Ingredients

- 1 cup diced Green /Yellow/ Red / Bell Peppers

- 1/2 cup diced Onions

- 1/4 cup of Black Olives

- 4 cups Spelt Pasta cooked

- 1 cup sliced Summer Squash/Zucchini

- 3/4 - 1 cup Garlic Sauce Alkaline

- 1/2 cup halved Cherry Tomatoes

Directions

1. In a wide bowl, combine all the ingredients until well combined, & enjoy your Pasta Salad.

4.2 Electric Ravioli Alkaline

Ingredients

Ravioli Filling

- 1/3 cup diced Onions,

- 1/3 cup diced Green Bell Pepper,

- 1 cup flour Garbanzo bean

- 1 tbsp. of Onion Powder

- 1 cup chopped Kale,

- 2 cups sliced Mushrooms,

- 1/3 cup diced Bell Pepper

- 1 Tomato

- 2 tsp. of Basil

- 1 tsp. of Ginger

- 2 tsp. of Oregano

- 1/2 tsp. Red Pepper Crushed

- 2 tsp. of Fennel Seeds

- 2 tsp. of Thyme

- 2 tsp. of Dill

- 1 tsp. of Sea Salt

- Food Processor

- 1/2 tsp. of Cayenne Powder

Dough

- 1/2 tsp. of Oregano

- 1/2 cup Flour Garbanzo Bean

- 1 1/2 cup of Spelt Flour

- 3/4 cup of Spring Water

- 1/2 tsp. of Basil

- 1 tsp. of Sea Salt

Cheese

- 1/2 tsp. of Cayenne

- 1/2 cup of Spring Water

- 1/2 cup Brazilian Nuts Soaked

- Blender

- 1 tsp. of Sea Salt

- 2 tsp. of Onion Powder

- 1/2 tsp. of Oregano

Directions

1. In the food processor, apply all the filling components excluding garbanzo flour, mix for 30 seconds, and blend in the flour just until incorporated.

2. Lightly brush the cast iron pan in grapeseed oil over moderate flame.

3. Spread the filling with the ravioli, cook on one side for 3-4 minutes, then turn & prepare for the next 3-4 minutes.

4. Place it away in a tub, split up the filling, and simmer for a couple more minutes.

5. In a mixer, put all the cheese ingredients and blend until creamy. If it is too dense, apply some spring water.

6. Pour all the ingredients of the dry dough into the food processor, combine for ten seconds, and steadily apply water and mix until the dough shapes into a shape. (If you don't have a blender, combine in a cup & knead before a ball form.)

7. Take 1/4 of dough into your palms, then roll the dough out on a floured area; add more flour if necessary.

8. Mix the cheese and fill the bowl full, and scoop the combination on one portion of dough approximately half an inch away.

9. Fold the dough over and pat the filling over, cut out the ravioli with the pastry cutter, and ensuring that every other ravioli is closed. (At this point, ravioli may be frozen and preserved for later.

10. Carry the spring water to a boil, apply a little oil and sea salt, and cook the ravioli about 4-6 mins.

11. Strain the ravioli until finished and encourage it to cool before eating.

12. Finish off and eat the ravioli with Tomato Sauce.

4.3 Electric Veggie Lasagna Alkaline

Ingredients

Tomato Sauce

- 1/2 tsp. of Cayenne Powder

- 12 Tomatoes Plum

- 1 tbsp. of Onion Powder

- 2 tsp. of Sea Salt

- 2 tsp. of Basil

- 1 tbsp. of Agave

- 2 tsp. of Oregano

"Meat" Alternative

- 1 cup Garbanzo Beans Cooked

- 2 tsp. of Oregano

- 2 cups Spelt Cooked

- 2 tbsp. of Onion Powder

- 1 tsp. of Fennel Powder

- 1 cup Yellow, Green, & Red Peppers

- 2 tsp. Basil

- 1/2 cup "Garlic" Sauce Alkaline

- 1 tbsp. of Sea Salt

- 1 cup Chopped Onions

Brazilian nut Cheese

- 1 cup of Spring Water

- 2 cups Brazilian Nuts Soaked

- 1 tsp. of Basil

- 1 tsp. of Sea Salt

- 1 tbsp. of Hemp Seeds

- 1 tsp. of Oregano

- 1 tbsp. of Onion Powder

Pasta

- Spelt Noodles Lasagna

Extras

- 9 x 13 Baking Dish Glass

- Grapeseed Oil

- White Mushrooms

- Zucchini

Directions

1. Mix all of the tomato sauce items together in a blender once well mixed.

2. On medium flame, connect to the saucepan & simmer, then cook the sauce over a low flame, stirring regularly about 2 hours or till thickened.

3. Mix garbanzo beans, spelt, & seasonings in the food processor till it's combined for the "meat" combination.

4. Light spray the pan using grapeseed oil over high heat and sauté the onions & peppers about 5 minutes.

5. In the pan, apply spelt/garbanzo bean blend & alkaline "garlic oil" and simmer about 10-12 mins or when it begins to brown.

6. In a blender, incorporate 1 cup spring & all the other cheese components and mix until blended. If it is too dense, apply 1/4 cup of water before you obtain the perfect consistency.

7. Place apart 1 cup tomato sauce, and add the remaining spelt/garbanzo bean blend into the leftover sauce and blend well.

8. Lengthwise, finely dice the mushrooms & zucchini. Instead of pasta, you can also make Lasagna from sliced zucchini as an alternative.

9. Start creating Lasagna in a glass dish by gently rubbing tomato sauce on the bottom of the plate. This is to prevent the pasta from sticking to the plate.

10. Add pasta, spelt/garbanzo blend, zucchini, mushrooms, cheese, then again with pasta. Till you have four layers of pasta, replicate this process.

11. Apply the spelt/garbanzo mix & cheese to the last surface of pasta, and pipe the leftover tomato sauce over the pasta.

12. Bake about 35-45 minutes at 350 ° F.

13. Enable 15 minutes to cool before serving & enjoy it!

4.4 Alkaline Sea Moss Apple Pie Smoothie

Ingredients

- 1 tbsp ginger fresh (optional)

- 1 heaping tbsp of Seamoss gel

- 2 cups of ice cubes

- 1 dash powdered Clove

- 2 cups apple juice fresh

Directions

1. Using a mixer to combine all the ingredients.

2. Blend until frothy & smooth.

3. Just serve!

4.5 Kale Smoothie Alkaline

Ingredients

- 1 apple2 cups coconut or spring water

- 2 handfuls of kale

- 1 thumb-sized ginger

- 1 tbsp gel of sea moss

- 1/4 cup of lime juice

- 1 cup of cucumber

Directions

1. Mix all the components together in a mixer.

2. Mix for 2 mins or till you have completely blended all the components in a smooth beverage.

3. Instantly serve or cool for afterward.

4. Place & refrigerate in the glass bottle—usage within 3 days.

4.6 Callaloo Smoothie Alkaline

Ingredients

- 1 large arugula bunch

- 1/4 cup of lime juice

- 1 large callaloo bunch

- 1 cup of cucumber

- 1 pear

- 1 thumb-sized ginger

- ¼ of honeydew

- 6 dates

- 1 tbsp gel of sea moss

- 2 cups coconut or spring water

Directions

1. Mix all the components together in a mixer.

2. Mix for 2 mins or till you have completely blended all the components in a smooth beverage.

3. Instantly serve or cool for afterward.

4. Place & refrigerate in the glass bottle—usage within 3 days.

4.7 Dandelion Smoothie Alkaline

Ingredients

- 1 handful of watercress
- 2 cups coconut or spring water
- 1/2 cup of blueberries
- 1 large dandelion greens bunch
- 1/4 cup of lime juice
- 6 dates
- 3 bananas
- 1 tbsp powdered burdock root
- 1 thumb-sized ginger

Directions

1. Mix all the components together in a mixer.

2. Mix for 2 mins or till you have completely blended all the components in a smooth beverage.

3. Instantly serve or cool for afterward.

4. Place & refrigerate in the glass bottle—usage within 3 days.

4.8 Hemp Mayo Alkaline

Ingredients

- 2 tbsp. of Grapeseed Oil
- 1 cup of Hemp Seeds
- 1/2 tsp. of Sea Salt
- 1 tbsp. of Onion Powder
- Stick Blender or Cup Blender
- 3/4 cup of Spring Water
- 1 tsp. of Lime Juice

Directions

1. Apply all the ingredients to the cup & blend until smooth for 30-60 seconds.

2. If you have very dense, add more water or even more seeds and condense if liquidy.

3. Stock and keep in the refrigerator in an air-tight jar.

4. Relish your Hemp Mayo!

4.9 Creamy Banana Pie Alkaline

Ingredients

Pie Mixture

- 7 oz. of Creamed Coconut
- 1/8 tsp. of Sea Salt
- 1 cup of hemp milk
- 6 – 8 Baby/Burro Bananas
- 3 – 4 tbsp. of Agave

Crust

- 1/4 tsp. of Sea Salt
- 1 1/2 cups Coconut Chips / Flakes Unsweetened
- 1 1/2 cups pitted Dates,
- 1/4 cup of Agave

Equipment

- Pie Dish
- Hand Mixer
- Food Processor

Directions

1. Put all crust components in a blender & combine for 20 to 30 seconds till a ball is created.

2. Top spring-form pot with the waxed sheet, then thinly spread the crust mixture out.

3. In a spring-form container, put thin slices bananas across them, then store them in the freezer.

4. Apply the pie blend components to a big bowl and combine until well mixed with your mixer.

5. Pour the pie mixture over the spring-form bowl, shake the sides and then cover it with foil & enable it to freeze about 3-4 hours.

6. Cover over coconut flakes, remove from the plate, and savor your Banana Pie!

4.10 Fruit Punch Alkaline

Ingredients

- 1 cup frozen Peaches,

- 1 cup frozen Blueberries,

- 1/2 to 1 cup Agave*

- Fine Strainer

- 1 cup frozen Cherries,

- 1 cup frozen Strawberries,

- 6 cups of Spring Water

- Ice

- Blender

Directions

1. In a blender, incorporate fruit, 1/2 cup of agave & 2 cups spring water & combine for around thirty seconds.

2. To extract unwanted seeds, pour the mixture through the strainer. (Optional step)

3. To a wide pitcher, put the combination, ice, and the remaining four cups water & combine.

4. Cherish your Fruit Punch.

4.11 Ginger Shot Alkaline

- **Ingredients**

- juice extractor

- 1 apple small

- 2 ounces ginger root fresh

Directions

1. Using a grater or spoon to scrape the ginger skin

2. Cut & add to the extractor for juice

3. Slice the apple and apply the ginger bits,

4. Juice

5. Add sliced apple & ginger to the mixer if you are using a processor.

6. Integrate 1-2 cups spring water

7. Mix well

8. Shear from a bag of cheesecloth or almond milk bag

9. Cherish the juice

P. S. As in spicy, this will be strongly intense & hot!

4.12 Alkaline Raw Tahini Butter

Ingredients

- food processor or blender

- 1 – 2 tbsp of grapeseed oil

- sesame seeds raw

Directions

1. To a processor cup, apply pure sesame seeds

2. Mix, so the paste is chunky.

3. Add oil

4. Mix with the honey.

5. Store in the fridge in glass jars

4.13 Alkaline Walnut Butter

Ingredients

- 1 tbsp raw agave (optional)

- 2 cups walnuts soaked

- 1/2 tsp sea salt

- 1 tsp avocado oil (optional)

Directions

1. For a minimum 1 hour or nightly, drench 2 cups walnuts in the spring water.

2. Water dump and dispose of.

3. To produce a roasted taste, bake the nuts in the oven at 350 ° about 10 minutes; this process is optional.

4. In a food processor, incorporate the nuts and combine until smooth, incorporating the rest of the materials.

5. Offer with spelt crackers or fruit

4.14 Alkaline Applesauce

Ingredients

- blender

- 3 tbsp agave

- 1/8 tsp cloves

- 3 cups apples peeled, chopped

- 1 tsp of Seamoss gel

- 1 tsp lime juice

- 1/2 cup of strawberries

- 1/8 tsp sea salt

- spring water

Directions

1. In addition to cloves, salt, lime juice, & agave, apply sliced apples to the blender.

2. Pulse to obtain the optimal quality using the blender.

3. Pulse through the strawberries just until combined.

4. If it doesn't mix well, apply 1 tablespoon spring water.

5. Serving and relax! Preserve the leftover food in the freezer.

4.15 Alkaline Brazilian nut Cheesecake

Ingredients

Cheesecake Mixture:

- 1/4 tsp. of Sea Salt

- 5-6 Dates

- 2 cups of Brazil Nuts

- 1/4 cup of Agave

- 1 1/2 cups Walnut Milk or Hemp Milk

- 1 tbsp. Gel of sea moss

- 2 tbsp. of lime Juice

Crust:

- 1/4 tsp. of Sea Salt

- 1/4 cup of Agave

- 1 1/2 cups of Coconut Flakes

- 1 1/2 cups of Dates

Toppings:

- sliced Strawberries,

- Blackberries

- sliced Raspberries,

- sliced mango,

- Blueberries

Tools:

- Parchment Paper

- Blender

- Food Processor

- 8-inch Pan spring-form

Directions

1. Put all the crust items and process for 20 seconds in the food processor.

2. In a springform pan filled with parchment spread the crust out.

3. Place the thin slices of mango around the pan's corners and stay in the freezer.

4. Apply all the ingredients in the cheesecake blend to the blender and process until blend.

5. Pour the mixture over the crust, wrap in foil & allow 3-4 hours to settle.

6. Remove the pan's shape, layer your toppings & enjoy!

Ensuring the leftovers are put in the fridge!

4.16 Alkaline Ginger Soup

Ingredients

- 1 cup red peppers diced
- 12-16 cups of spring water
- 4-6 Leaves of Soursop
- 3 tbsp onion powder
- 2 cups kale chopped
- 1 cup onions diced
- 1 cup cubed zucchini
- 4 tsp sea salt
- 1 cup cubed summer squash
- 1 cup green peppers diced
- 1 tbsp minced fresh ginger,
- 2 cups cubed chayote squash
- 1 tbsp basil
- 1 cup Quinoa

- 1/4 tsp cayenne (optional)

- 1 tbsp oregano

Directions

1. Rinse the leaves, rip them in half, and put them in a wide stockpot containing 4 cups of spring water.

2. With a cap on the kettle, boil the leaves about 15-20 mins.

3. Extract the leaves from the broth.

4. The remaining ingredients are added.

5. Add 8 cups of spring water.

6. Combine all the ingredients, replace the cap, and simmer for 30-45 minutes over medium heat. (If you do not use quinoa, more time will be required.)

4.17 Alkaline Zucchini Bacon

Ingredients

- 2 tbsp. of Agave

- 1/4 cup of Date Sugar

- 2-3 Zucchini

- 1 tbsp. of Sea Salt Smoked

- 1/2 tsp. of Cayenne Powder

- 1 tbsp. of Onion Powder

- 1/4 cup of Spring Water

- Potato Peeler/ Mandoline

- 1 tsp. of Liquid Smoke

- Grapeseed Oil

- 1/2 tsp. of Ginger Powder

- Parchment Paper

Directions

1. In a saucepan, incorporate all the ingredients and simmer on low heat until they are dissolved.

2. Chop finishes off the zucchini and makes strips with a potato peeler.

3. Toss the zucchini with the saucepan ingredients in a wide cup, then enable it to marinate for 30-60 minutes. There is no need for more water since it will emerge from zucchini.

4. On a baking sheet, put parchment paper then slightly brush with the grapeseed oil.

5. Cover the marinated strips with the baking sheets, then bake at 400 ° F for 10 minutes.

6. Flip the strips of zucchini over & cook for the next 3-4 minutes, then let it cool off.

7. Cook for another few minutes or sear in a finely oil-coated pan for 30 seconds if you like to make any of the strips more crispy.

8. Enjoy your Bacon with Zucchini!

4.18 Alkaline Biscuits

Ingredients

- 1 tsp. of Sea Salt

- 3/4 cup Coconut Milk/Quinoa Milk

- Cup /Cookie Cutter

- 1/4 cup of Grapeseed Oil

- 2 cups of Spelt Flour

Directions

1. Mix all the components in a bowl together before they have shaped together into a ball.

2. Stretch out 1'' thick dough, then turn the dough over the highest part of itself & spread out once again.

3. Slice out the biscuits using a cookie cutter after turning over the dough around 4-5 times.

4. On a baking sheet, place the biscuits. (Optional parchment paper)

5. Bake about 18-20 mins at 350 ° F.

6. Enable it to cool down and have fun.

4.19 Alkaline Teff Sausage

Ingredients

- 1/4 cup onions diced

- 1 1/2 cups Teff Grain cooked

- 1 tbsp. diced Red Peppers,

- 2 tsp. of Ground Sage

- 1 tbsp. diced Green Peppers,

- 1 tsp. of Oregano

- 1/2 cup of Chickpea Flour

- 1 tbsp. of Onion Powder

- 1/2 tsp. of Dill

- 1 tsp. of Fennel Powder

- 1/2 tsp. Red Pepper Crushed

- 1 tsp. of Sea Salt

- Grapeseed Oil

- Skillet

- 1 tsp. of Basil

- Mixing Bowl

Directions

1. Sauté the peppers & onions in around 1 tbsp of grapeseed oil about 2-3 mins over medium-high flame.

2. Lastly, apply the rest of the ingredients & sautéed veggies to chickpea flour in a wide bowl and combine well.

3. Add 1-2 teaspoons grapeseed oil to the skillet over medium heat.

4. Shape the teff blend forming patties & cook it on each side for 3 minutes, until crunchy.

5. Cherish your sausage of Teff!

4.20 Alkaline French toast

Ingredients

- 1/2 cup Flour Garbanzo Bean
- Grapeseed Oil
- 1/2 tsp. of Ground Cloves
- 3/4 cup Walnut Milk /Hemp Milk
- 1/4 cup of Spring Water
- Spelt Bread
- 2 tbsp. of Agave
- 1/4 tsp. of Sea Salt
- Strawberries sliced (optional)
- 1/4 tsp. of Ginger Powder

Directions

1. In a wide container, blend together all the ingredients until well combined.

2. Pour the batter into the long jar and allow the bread to steep about 5-10 mins, midway through tossing the bread.

3. Lightly oil the skillet using grapeseed oil on a moderate flame and steam about 3-4 mins or till brown.

4. Round off with agave and strawberries, and enjoy!

Chapter 5: Herb Approach to Cure Herpes

This chapter includes a detailed list of all the herbs along with the parts of the herb that is allowed to be consumed. These are the herbs that help to alkalize the body because it is believed that the acidic body will lead to the occurrence of other diseases. There are also other diseases that are cured with the help of these herbs. Single herb does not perform a specific function but is almost helpful for the overall health of the individual.

5.1 Oregano

In the mint family, oregano is indeed a popular herb that is generally known only for its extremely impressive healing properties. Antiviral effects are given by the plant products that include carvacrol.

Both oregano oil and extracted carvacrol decreased murine norovirus (MNV) behavior within 15 min of exposure in a test-tube sample.

MNV is particularly infectious in humans and is the main source of stomach flu. It is somewhat close to real norovirus and is used in research experiments as it is extremely difficult to produce human norovirus in laboratory environments.

The antiviral activity mostly against HSV-1; rotavirus, a frequent cause of diarrhea in children and babies; & respiratory virus (RSV), which induces respiratory problems, has been shown to exhibit oregano oil & carvacrol.

5.2 Sage

Sage, also a part of the mint tribe, is an herbal plant that has traditionally been used to cure viral infections in conventional medicine.

The antiviral effects of sage are often due to the safficinolide & sage-one compounds present in the plant's stems & leaves.

Test-tube testing shows that this herb can combat HIV-1, which can contribute to AIDS. In one analysis, by keeping that virus from accessing target cells, sage extract greatly prevented HIV operation.

Sage which have been shown to fight with HSV-1 & Indiana vesiculovirus, which infects livestock such as cows, pigs, & horses.

5.3 Basil

Many types of basil can combat some viral infections, including that of the sweet & holy variants.

For instance, test-tube research reported that the sweet basil abstract exhibited a profound impact toward enterovirus, hepatitis B, & herpes viruses, involving compounds such as apigenin & ursolic acid.

It has been proven that holy basil, otherwise recognized as tulsi, enhances immunity, which can help combat infectious diseases.

Significantly improved amounts of helper T-cells & natural killer, which are both immune cells that help support & preserve the body against viral infections, were combined with 300 mg holy basil concentrate in a 4-week sample in 24 normal individuals.

Studies say that tulsi should also be used to cure the notorious herpes outbreak, a communicable disease triggered by the HSV/human herpesvirus, while it tends to relieve mild infections. The virus stays inactive in the process for life until the individual gets infected and may trigger breakouts during stressful times. What makes it more humiliating for the patient is the cold sores across the mouth are triggered by HSV-1, which really is oral herpes.

There is no remedy for the virus, and antiviral drugs such as famciclovir, acyclovir, & valacyclovir are used in standard therapy approaches for herpes contamination. But the prospect of curing herpes using a systemic method, primarily using holy basil, is now being investigated by researchers. Do you realize the Tulsi has these beneficial effects?

In research reported in African Journal, scientists explored the antiviral efficacy of dichloromethane & tulsi methanol extracts against HSP in particular. The analysis showed that tulsi had such an inhibitory impact at different levels in the production of the virus on herpes pathogen.

How would basil be used for HSV prevention?

Tulsi is indeed a body's natural booster that reinforces the defences of your body. It may be used either as a prophylactic or a curative step. Routinely sipping a decoction of tulsi could improve your immunity to combat infections. Or, it is necessary to topically add a paste produced from the leaves & blossoms from tulsi to the location of the herpes outbreak.

5.4 Fennel

Fennel is a plant flavored with liquorice that may combat such pathogens.

A test-tube analysis found that there were good antiviral impacts of fennel extract toward herpes viruses & type 3 parainfluenza (PI-3), which triggers cattle respiratory problems.

Moreover, the key ingredient of fennel oil, trans-anethole, has been shown to have powerful antiviral activity toward herpes viruses.

Fennel will also improve the immune system & reduce inflammation, and can also help against viral infections, as per animal studies.

5.5 Peppermint

It is understood that peppermint has potent antiviral effects and is widely applied to teas, oils, and tinctures intended to cure viral infections naturally.

Its leaves & essential oils include active ingredients that have antiviral & anti-inflammatory function, which include menthol & rosmarinic acid.

Peppermint-leaf decoction demonstrated effective antiviral action toward respiratory virus (RSV) in a test-tube sample and dramatically decreased inflammatory substance concentrations.

5.6 Sambucus

Sambucus is a species of elderly plants. Elderberries are produced into a range of items that are used to spontaneously cure respiratory illnesses such as fever & common cold, such as medicines & elixirs.

Research in mice confirmed that condensed elderberry concentrate inhibited the development of influenza viruses and activated the reaction of the immune system.

What's more, elderberry extracts have been shown to greatly alleviate upper respiratory issues induced through viral infections in a study of 4 trials in 180 adults.

5.7 Astragalus

Astragalus is common in Chinese traditional medicine as the flowering herb. It has Astragalus polysaccharide

(APS) that has important insulin-improving & antiviral effects.

Test-tube & animal tests indicate that herpes, hepatitis C, & avian influenza viruses are combated by astragalus.

Including test-tube experiments indicate that APS may shield astrocyte cells in humans from herpes infection, the most common form of cells in CNS.

5.8 Ginger

Ginger goods are common natural remedies, including tonics, teas, & lozenges, and with good purpose. Characterized by its high content of powerful plant compounds, ginger is shown to have remarkable antiviral efficacy.

Test-tube study indicates that its extract, which is similar to human norovirus, has antiviral activity toward RSV, avian influenza, & (FCV) feline calicivirus.

In addition, various ginger compounds, such as gingerol & zingerone, have already been found to impede viral replication & avoid the entrance of viruses into host cells.

Ginger's health advantages include the capacity to decrease inflammation and kill microbes and viruses.

Ginger often lowers inflammation, soothes the throat, improves flora, and treats elevated blood pressure in the digestive tract.

Ginger, especially in broad and distilled amounts, maybe very hot for certain individuals. Select the proper number that can be supported by you.

Health Advantages

Ginger is indeed the underground herb of Zingiber officinale or rhizome. For thousands of years, herbalists used these ginger being part of natural medicine because of its usefulness in the management of sore stomachs, diarrhea, and nausea.

In order to cure arthritis, colic, diarrhea, cold or flu, flu-like symptoms, vomiting, and uncomfortable menstrual cycles, herbalists have often used ginger.

The medicinal powers of gingers are extracted from volatile oils, which include gingerols & shogaols.

1. Ginger increases saliva production, thereby making it very easy to swallow.

2. by behaving like blood pressure drugs labeled "calcium channel blockers," ginger lowers elevated blood pressure.

The influx of calcium towards heart cells & blood vessels is regulated by ginger, thus lower blood pressure.

3. It inhibits the production of prostaglandins, the pro-inflammatory substances in the body, and thereby decreases systemic inflammation. The latest research has shown that genes in the body that encode the molecules found in persistent inflammation may be blocked or deactivated by the ginger extract. It seems that shogaol phytonutrients present in ginger have their anti-inflammatory value.

4. Ginger minimizes osteoarthritis pressure.

5. Motion sickness is minimized by ginger: nausea, vomiting, and a general sense of queasy. This advantage tends to be provided by gingerol phytonutrients from ginger.

6. Ginger has properties that are anti-bacterial. Extracts of ginger stems, viz. ethyl acetate n-hexane, & soxhlet extracts possess anti-bacterial activities over coliform bacillus, epidermidis staphylococcus, and viridian streptococcus.

7. Ginger has antiviral qualities.

5.9 Dandelion

Dandelions have been investigated for various medicinal uses, including possible antiviral impact, but are generally known as weeds.

The test-tube study suggests that HIV, hepatitis B, & influenza may be combated through dandelion.

In addition, one test tube analysis indicated that the development of dengue that triggers dengue fever was blocked by extract of dandelion. Signs, including high fever, vomiting, & muscle pain, are caused by this illness, which may be lethal.

5.10 Hydrangea Herb

Root Benefits

Hydrangea is indeed a genus comprising 70 to 75 species in the family of plants known as hydrangeaceae, which has various properties based mostly on species.

The hydrangea plant included in Chinese medicine is Chang Shan (Dichroa Root or Dichroa febrifuga), which is indigenous to East Asia.

The typical hydrangea indigenous to America is Hydrangea arborescens (wild Sevens barks, hydrangea).

Hydrangea root compounds have been used to cure auto-immune diseases & remove bacteria, have been used as a diuretic & blood cleanser, and have been used for the prevention of bladder & kidney stones to reduce calcification.

Parasitic Infections

The anti-parasitic trait is also accountable for the febriugine substance in the hydrangea root of Chang Shan. Febriugine interferes with the aminoacylation mechanism that helps individuals to synthesize the proteins human beings need to survive, destroying malaria from the bloodstream efficiently.

Kidney Stones and Calcification

Thanks to its capacity to remove calcium compounds by its soapy activity, the Hydrangea root genus, like Hydrangea arborescens, is known as a lithotriptic herb.

Calcification is desired in bones and teeth, but soft tissue calcification is undesired & disrupts normal cellular functions.

In herbal medicine, Hydrangea root is used to disintegrate calcium deposits in the kidneys & bladder and, in general, to dissolve soft tissue calcification.

It is necessary to decalcify soft tissue since it enables beneficial components for viruses as well as other toxic materials to reach and clean cells.

Hydrangea produces hydrangin (skimmetin), the organic phytochemical solvent that has been active in the capacity of hydrangea to remove calcium deposits.

General Benefits

Swollen prostate glands have been handled with Hydrangea leaf. The anti-inflammatory effects of Hydrangea derive from its capacity to suppress pro-inflammatory substances like prostaglandin E2, nitric oxide, & necrosis factor-alpha (TNF-alpha).

Hydrangea root itself is a diuretic which cleanses the urinary tract by rising urination. To make sure that you stay hydrated, it is necessary to consume around 3/4 -1 gallon water per day. Hydrangea is a plant producing phosphorus, iron, calcium, magnesium, potassium, & sulfur that is high in minerals. Hydrangea root even produces elevated amounts of cell-damage-protective kaempferol, flavonoids, saponin, quercetin, & volatile oil.

5.11 Anamu

Guinea hen weed is an herb common in Jamaica and has historically been used to treat diseases such as cancer. Petiveria alliacea L is the botanical term for Guinea hen weed, and its success has contributed to many research studies on the herb being performed.

These experiments also contributed to the realization that a significant cause for its curing powers was one of the plant's metabolites. In its cancer combat potential, this main metabolite named dibenzyl trisulfide performs a big role.

Recent research has introduced a more impressive property to the long list of medicinal benefits of anamu. An analysis found that the dibenzyl trisulfide metabolite inhibits the HIV-1 reverse transcriptase protein.

HIV) produces an enzyme that reads and recodes the sequence as a DNA sequence of the viral RNA sequence of that has reached a cell. This makes it impossible for the immune system since it lies right underneath the radar of the immune system to better track and destroy the virus.

The enzyme recoding the sequence is named "reverse transcriptase," and the analysis shows that dibenzyl trisulfide prevents the capacity of HIV to recode HIV's viral RNA into DNA.

By preventing reverse transcriptase protein from recoding the viral RNA into DNA, medications such as azidothymidine (AZT) have been used to fight the dissemination of HIV in the body. The industry will use technology to synthesize the guinea hen weed's reverse transcriptase impairing characteristics.

Our socialized paradigms would prevent all of us from reaching for the soothing plants that are a gift from "The Harmony" of creation and nature behind our noses. To keep us safe, we have to get back in contact with nature & use what that has given for us for free.

5.12 Elderberry

Elderberry, also recognized for Sambucus Nigra, has been used for thousands of years in alternative medicine to combat cold & flu problems. Elderberries have historically been used to treat fever and colds, and now experimental evidence has proven that their antiviral & antioxidant effects are the explanation for their efficacy. Analysis has shown that by attaching to virus & preventing it from accessing host cells, elderberry has been successful toward flu infections such as H1N1.

5.13 Sea Moss

102 minerals are provided by 92 of the bodies. Some of its several advantages include potassium chloride source, advantages: teeth, eczema, psoriasis, colds & flu, muscles, heart, radiation exposure, cancer rehabilitation, sunburn, dysentery, rashes, heart, bones, diabetes, thyroid, & weight loss.

5.14 Nopal cactus

In powder form has been used to suppress blood pressure, repair wounds, and lower cholesterol levels. The anti-inflammatory and antioxidant effects of the plant have been verified by tests. Many of the other supposed advantages include the ability to assist in weight control, avoidance of disease, enhancing skin wellbeing, controlling and increasing nutrition, strengthening the immune system, creating solid muscles, reduction of sleeplessness & reducing increased inflammation of the body, strengthening metabolism.

5.15 Cocolmeca

Cleanses the liver & is anti-inflammatory, manages diseases, ulcers of the stomach and digestive tract, and cleanses the intestines. This incredible plant, when the blood is compromised by toxicity like Sickle Cell, has the potential to repair healthy blood. It offers advantages like anti-bacterial, anti-microbial, antifungal, and anti-inflammatory & rheumatism, sexual impotence, skin conditions such as acne, & records the advantages of shrinking cysts & burning body fat.

5.16 Horsetail

Hair, Brittle bones, gingivitis, teeth, tonsillitis, acne, diabetes, rheumatic diseases, edema, rashes, itchy skin, frostbite wounds, chilblains, cracked and sore feet, and ulcers are handled by horsetail. Horsetail often decreases inflammation, prevents tumors, strengthens the immune system, helps to defend the kidneys and intellect. Toxic aluminium is extracted from the body to avoid Alzheimer's disease.

5.17 Baobob

It's a substance from the seed of the Baobob tree. It is among the five best alkaline fruits, filled with vitamin C 33 percent, rich in fiber, suppresses appetite, decreases inflammation, due to its high fiber content, ideal for pregnant females because it helps regulate blood sugar, prebiotics promotes healthy digestive health & feels of fullness as it helps shape collagen in babies and promotes the healthy immune system. Promotes skin that is safe. It can be found in smoothies, porridge, salads, and tea.

5.18 Gotu Kola

Promotes a balanced cardiovascular and circulatory system, replenishes the natural energy store of the body, increases performance and attention, enhances the immune system throughout challenging times, regenerates the nervous system, enhances clearer skin, helps smooth cellulite & calms varicose veins.

5.19 Fenugreek

Lack of flavor, anemia, fever, dandruff, digestive problems, biliousness, respiratory disorders, oral ulcers, diabetes, sore throat, inflammation, wounds, & insomnia are the health advantages of fenugreek. It is effective in lactation & tends to boost digestion & quality of the scalp. It is also seen that levels of cholesterol are lowered, and cardiac function is preserved, while at the same time improving the immune system & defending against influenza and different infections. A sweet craving is also suppressed by fenugreek.

5.20 Guaco

Preferred as the anti-inflammatory in Brazil. Pain relievers & antispasmodics. Ulcers, Intestinal swelling, arthritis & rheumatism. For eczema, neuralgia, wounds, & pruritis, a leaf decoction may be administered directly.

5.21 Chaparral

STD's nervous system disorders, chickenpox, snakebite pain, parasite diseases, obesity, used for cancer, arthritis, UTI, tuberculosis, may also be consumed for detoxifying or even as an elixir for blood purifier

5.22 Arnica

Eczema, Enhance wound recovery, Sore nostrils, Tendon or cartilage discomfort, Minimize inflammation & swelling, Ease injuries irritations, Soothe and cure bruises as well as sprains, Ulcers, Arthritis, Acne, Chapped lips, Burns,

5.23 Yellow Dock

Pain & swelling (irritation) of the nasal cavity, Rashes, Skin diseases, Respiratory tract, Scurvy, STD, dermatitis, Psoriasis (constipation) Avoid or reduce cancer development, Tonic, Toothpaste, Bacterial infections care, Yellow Dock-Obstructive jaundice, Enlarged lymph, Constant sweating, Laxative,

5.24 Stinging Nettle

Increased spleen, anemia, hypertension, astringent, enlarged prostate, blood washing, bowel leakage, cancer, digestive system, diarrhea, diabetes, diuretic (joint disease), dysentery, general tonic, eczema, urinary tract, gout, hemorrhage, loss of hair (alopecia), urination, hay fever, pneumonia, kidney stones, irritable bladder,

5.25 Chaga

Dense superfood foods, decreasing blood pressure, cholesterol, battling the disease, preventing aging, inflammation allows reducing blood sugar in the immune system. Vitamin D, B-complex, amino acids, potassium, fiber, copper, zinc, iron, manganese, calcium and magnesium, complex vitamins,

5.26 Sencha

The potential to decrease the likelihood of cancer, avoid infectious disorders, lower blood pressure, regulate cholesterol levels, help in weight reduction, strengthen the immune system, boost vitality and promote cognitive function is filled with several advantages.

5.27 Ashwagandha

Improves the protection of the thyroid & adrenal glands, decreases depression and exhaustion, protects from stomach ulcers, anti-cancer, anti-tumor, anti-inflammatory, help for the central nervous system, increased resilience. Memory and comprehension are strengthened, immunity is boosted, mitochondrial capacity & energy levels are raised. Reducing fear, raising muscle strength.

5.28 Lavender

Reduces distress and mental tension, defends against diabetes, enhances cognitive activity, cures wounds and injuries, preserves the complexion of the face, speeds down the aging process, enhances sleep, relieves headaches and discomfort, improves blood pressure, boosts digestion and digestive wellbeing, helps reduce hair loss, increases urinary production.

5.29 Kalawalla

It helps to stabilize the blood cleanser, immune system, neuroprotective, skin cells, decreases irritation, and relieves itchy skin, redness, and flaking of scalp accumulation. Used to help overcome auto-immune conditions like Lupus & MS. Natural sunscreen decreases phlegm.

5.30 Blue Vervain

It has antimalarial diuretic properties. Traditionally used in medications for the prevention of menstrual cramps, anti-inflammatory drugs to improve milk intake of breastfeeding mothers. Nervous symptoms, including fatigue, anxiety & restlessness, are mainly used to treat

5.31 Bladder wrack

Super & hypoactive thyroids aid with the maximum Iodine level than any other plants. Obesity is treated, digestion is boosted, bones are enhanced, movement is enhanced, premature aging is avoided, cancer incidence is decreased, and cardiac wellbeing is enhanced. Vision protection & lowers swelling.

5.32 Canessa

Generally used for discomfort, including muscle distress, fatigue, rheumatoid arthritis, menstrual cramps, gout, and spinal disorder termed ankylosing spondylitis, it is used to manage HIV / AIDS when mixed with Sarsaparilla as well as other herbs. Prevents heart disease, anti-inflammatory, aids for anemia, asthma, digestive issues, depression, menstrual disorders, acne & jaundice—a perfect supply of iron.

5.33 Root for Burdock

Antioxidants, one of the strongest blood purifiers, cure or avoid tumors, minimize pain, cure and/or eliminate bacteria, and alleviate stiffness and arthritis deposits in the joints. For cuts, burns, and skin disorders, it may be used externally.

5.34 Root of Rhubarb

It has 11 tremendous health benefits, especially instances of reducing Alzheimer's, anti-aging, anti-inflammatory, strengthening muscles, lowering cholesterol levels, increasing digestive wellbeing, minimizing the risk of cancer, and curing constipation.

5.35 Palmetto Saw

The berries of this plant are being used for prostate cancer, hypertension, hair loss, prostate shrinking, cancer cell prevention, and testosterone regulation medicinally often used to purify the system & reduce the appetite for alcoholic drinks.

5.36 Moss Sea (Irish)

It has anti-microbial, anti-inflammatory & laxative effects, soothes colds, coughs & bronchitis, gastric ulcers, tuberculosis, & stomach disorders with swollen mucous membranes. Seamoss helps the protection of joints and eyes. It acts as a natural mineral aid with a broad variety of nutrients (92).

5.37 Black Walnut

If combined with herbs like Chickweed, Mullein, Cascara Sagrada, & Yellow Dock, to mention a few, removing mucus from the body is quite effective.

5.38 The Wormwood

Anti-bacterial, anti-inflammatory, improves hunger, treats anti-oxidant, anti-microbial disease, and manages numerous stomach conditions and issues regarding the gall bladder. Wormwood is now often used to prevent gastrointestinal spasms.

5.39 Powdered Reishi Mushroom

Considered to be one of the best tonics and a vitality driver. Reishi mushroom can also be used to reduce tension, to support the heart, and to normalize blood pressure with anti-oxidants. Antihistamine, shielding the kidneys, anti-carcinogenic, minimizing chemotherapy side effects, anti-bacterial. It triggers the immune system and, in particular, prevents HIV virus replication. It soothes nerves & relieves sleeplessness.

5.40 Sarsaparilla

Of all in the botanical setting, this herb has the maximum iron content. It has anti-ulcer, anti-inflammatory, anti-oxidant, diaphoretic & diuretic anti-cancer properties. The capacity to attach with contaminants to promote their elimination from the body and blood has also been accredited to Sarsaparilla. It has been used in herbal medicine to cure skin disorders such as leprosy, psoriasis, rheumatoid arthritis, knee discomfort, fatigue, colds, & impotency.

5.41 A Red Clover

Such an herb helps to eliminate contaminants from the lymphatic system, alleviates effects of menopause fatigue, helps preserve a good appearance of the skin, lowers cholesterol, enhances cardiac condition, promotes immune, and helps improve hair follicles—prevention of cancer, bronchitis, sexually transmitted infections, breast pain, and PMS relief.

5.42 Chickweed

It increases drainage and helps reduce infection and leakage from the lungs, intestines, and stomach. It tends to liquefy and expel mucus from the respiratory system, helps to eliminate body fat, and can be used as an acne cleanser.

Chapter 6: Dr. Sebi Products to Cure Herpes Definitely

In this chapter, the products that mainly focuses on the immune system and how to reduce the inflammation are mentioned. These are basically the herbal teas or nutritional supplements. They are being used widely for the betterment of health and well-being. As all the diseases are the outcome of mucus, acidity, and a weak immune system, these products will help you to improve these specific areas of well-being.

6.1 Therapeutic Compounds

The African Bio-Mineral Treatment Method studies and recognizes the mechanisms of sickness, not only the effects. In addition, it found that mucus is the source of the disorder. Inside the body, where mucus has been collected, an illness may appear. While the natural food compounds of the vegetation cells were engineered to remove mucus from a specific region of the body, it is often important to clean the body as a whole. The nature in which they function to purify & nourish the whole body is what renders the compounds special.

We have been active in restoring pathologies through this method. As the herbs included have such a natural background, 14 days after they have been initially taken, the compounds also unleash their cleaning properties.

Adhering to the therapeutic recommendations given by Dr. Sebi is an equally significant feature of the African Bio-Mineral treatment. In order to maintain optimum wellness, our herbal compounds acting in combination with dietary improvements would give the body the correct climate. Also, please notice that if a meal is not mentioned in these sections, you are highly encouraged not to consume it. In addition, we notice that consuming a gallon of water recommended by Dr. Sebi every day tends to achieve the African Bio-Mineral Treatment most valuable outcomes.

6.2 Dr. Sebi's Immune Support Herbal Tea

Ingredients

- Elderberry

Directions

Heat two cups of purified water and apply 11/2 tablespoons of herbal tea from Dr. Sebi's Immune Help. Simmer for 15 minutes, roughly. Enable it to cool off. Strain. You can drink twice a day.

Dr. Sebi has added the organic antioxidant, called elderberry, to Immune Strength Herbal Tea. Elderberries could help minimize mucous membrane swelling, including sinus swelling, and alleviate nasal and antiviral inflammation & anti-cancer effects. Helping to improve the immune response is ideal. Elderberry will also minimize cholesterol, boost vision, coughs, sore throats, colds, pneumonia, diseases of bacteria and viruses, and some respiratory disorders. Protects from diseases of autoimmune nature. Elderberry often produces flavonoids possessing antioxidant effects, which may help protect the cells in the body from becoming harmed.

6.3 Energy Booster

Ingredients

- Muicle

Directions

Boil two cups of purified water and apply 1 1/2 tbsp of the Energy Booster from Dr. Sebi. Simmer for 15 minutes, roughly. Enable it to cool off. Strain. You can drink twice a day.

How does it help?

The Energy Booster from Dr. Sebi is directly targeted at improving your body as well as its activity levels. It boosts the amounts of iron in the bloodstream, which brings enough oxygen in the body throughout the haemoglobin of RBC so that cells can create energy. Muicle herb could be used as a blood purifier because of its antioxidant qualities, detoxifying advantages, and performance. To this day, as a component of everyday practice to become more energized than ever, many appreciate the advantages of this potent herb.

6.4 Bio-Ferro Tonic

Ingredients

- Burdock Root

- Cocolmeca

- Chaparral

- Elderberry

- Yellow dock

How does it help?

Bio Ferro blends the right components to have the most potent and powerful purifier and blood nourisher. Yellow dock is indeed an organic herb that is used as a bitter digestive for individuals with weak digestion. The root of Yellow dock, particularly for the liver, is a blood cleanser & overall detoxifier. The root of the yellow dock stimulates the development of bile, which aids digestion, especially of fats. To further clear the remaining waste from the digestive tract, it may promote bowel movement; it also improves the frequent urination to further eradicate contaminants.

6.5 Cleansing Package (Small)

How does it help?

Chelation2, Viento & Bio Ferro compose Small Cleaning Kit. This cleaning product is built at the cell level to cleanse & renourish the body.

The kit will help you get rid of mucus, contaminants, and acids from the body that collect in the system. It would, therefore, nourish & purify blood & add a safe condition to the whole body.

6.6 Bromide+ Capsules

Ingredients

- Bladder wrack
- Irish Seamoss

How does it help?

For the thyroid gland and bones. For people suffering from poor breath, lung ailments, lung conditions, dysentery, it is good. Bromide Plus serves as the organic diuretic, reduces the appetite, controls the intestines, and supports the digestive tract as a whole. In the total digestive tract, bromide Plus is beneficial. Bladder wrack is the seaweed that is distributed on the Pacific, Atlantic, and Baltic coasts. It is known as iodine's initial source. Bladder wrack is high in bromine, beta-carotene, alginic, potassium, & mannitol.

6.7 Green Food

Ingredients

- Bladder wrack
- Nettle
- Nopal
- Tila

How does it help?

The multi-Mineral formula is produced with African herbs that supply the whole body with chlorophyll-rich food. It promotes improved wellness and nourishment, generally. As an effective anti-inflammatory plant, Ortiga is well recognized. Treating kidney diseases, illnesses of the urinary tract (large prostate, urination at night, irregular urination, irritable bladder & painful urination), diseases of the gastrointestinal tract, and disorders of the locomotor system, cardiovascular system, rheumatism, influenza, hemorrhage, & gout. As a blood purifier, it is often successful, and low circulation is handled. Ortiga has also been used to relieve signs of allergies, such as hay fever in particular.

6.8 Viento

Ingredients

- Bladder wrack
- Chaparral
- Hombre Grande
- Hierba-Del Sapo
- Valeriana

How does it help?

Viento is a revitalizer, cleanser & energizer. As an effective antioxidant, Chaparral has been described. Chaparral has been used by Native Americans to cure different illnesses such as infectious disorder, snake bite, chickenpox, and discomfort from arthritis. Chaparral is a perfect cure for liver health, blood filtering, immune improvement, weight reduction, and general well-being thanks to its potent antioxidant possession. It is also used to address issues of metabolism, like cramps & gas, and disorders of the respiratory tract.

6.9 Iron Plus

Ingredients:

- Bugleweed
- Chaparral
- Hombre Grande
- Elderberry
- Palo Guaco
- Blue Vervain

How does it help?

Purifies all of the methods. As an effective antioxidant, Chaparral has been described. Chaparral has been used by Native Americans to cure different illnesses such as infectious disorder, snake bite, chickenpox, and discomfort from arthritis. Chaparral is a perfect cure for liver health, blood filtering, immune improvement, weight reduction, and general well-being thanks to its potent antioxidant capacity. It is also used to address issues of metabolism, such as cramps & gas, & disorders of the respiratory tract.

6.10 Nerve / Stress Relief Tea

Ingredients

- Chamomile

Directions

Add 1 tbsp of Herbal Tea and heat two cups of purified water. Steep, strain & drink during the evening for 10 to 15 minutes.

How does it help?

Chamomile tea from Dr. Sebi offers a gentle sleeping and calming boost. Chamomile is a moderate sedative that may lead to attitude change. It allows the muscles to calm and reduce impulsivity. Chamomile, while offering a powerful anti-inflammatory, anti-bacterial & antioxidant for basic everyday usage, can also offer relief from IBS and many stomach issues.

6.11 Stomach Relief Tea

Ingredients:

- Cuachalalate

Directions

Boil the purified water in two cups and apply 1 1/2 teaspoons of Digestive Relaxation Tea. Boil for 15 minutes, roughly. Enable it to cool off. Pressure. You can drink twice a day.

How does it help?

Cuachalalate, a popular herb being used by Central Americans for timely relief of certain stomach & gastric discomfort, including gastric ulcers, stomach cancer, and kidney illness, is produced from Dr. Sebi's herbs. Many can often receive comfort from urinary & renal discomfort & suffering from mouth infections, gastric ulcers, or superficial cuts, which is an ancient medicinal injection.

Conclusion

With the advancement in every field of life, we have become dependent on the shortcuts and immediate solutions to everything, whether it's a disease or any other issue. However, Dr. Sebi's diet and recommendations encourage you to move towards nature as close as possible. Nature is a healing entity in itself. For the centuries, herbs are being used for their enormous health benefits. They are used for common to most severe diseases. Dr. Sebi has provided with the list of herbs, and he also formulated certain ratios to use them as a supplement. His supplements are available to fulfill the needs of the human body with respect to nutrients and minerals. Along with that, food items are also specified for the one who is going to adapt his diet methods. Although this diet completely inhibits the protein intake, it surely covers up for the required amount of protein from other sources. As any sort of illness or disease arises from mucus accumulation in the human body and level of acidity, it is essential; to maintain these levels in the human body so that it can function properly, and hence it results in longevity. To attain the maximum level of health and well-being, one should get these supplements and follow the diet prescribed by Dr. Sebi. You can start by baby steps towards adopting this lifestyle, and it will shift everything for you in return.

CPSIA information can be obtained
at www.ICGtesting.com
Printed in the USA
LVHW100955180121
676360LV00041B/889